ONE HEALTH

From **A**IDS to **Z**ika

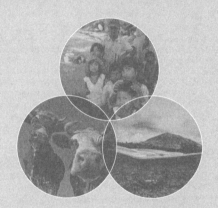

Richard Riegelman, MD, MPH, PhD
Professor and Founding Dean
Milken Institute School of Public Health
The George Washington University
Washington, DC

Brenda Kirkwood, MPH, DrPH
School of Public Health
University at Albany, State University of New York
Albany, New York

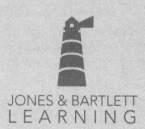

JONES & BARTLETT
LEARNING

World Headquarters
Jones & Bartlett Learning
5 Wall Street
Burlington, MA 01803
978-443-5000
info@jblearning.com
www.jblearning.com

Jones & Bartlett Learning books and products are available through most bookstores and online booksellers. To contact Jones & Bartlett Learning directly, call 800-832-0034, fax 978-443-8000, or visit our website, www.jblearning.com.

Substantial discounts on bulk quantities of Jones & Bartlett Learning publications are available to corporations, professional associations, and other qualified organizations. For details and specific discount information, contact the special sales department at Jones & Bartlett Learning via the above contact information or send an email to specialsales@jblearning.com.

Production Credits
VP, Executive Publisher: David D. Cella
Publisher: Michael Brown
Associate Editor: Lindsey Mawhiney Sousa
Production Editor: Vanessa Richards
Senior Marketing Manager: Sophie Fleck Teague
Manufacturing and Inventory Control Supervisor: Amy Bacus
Composition: Integra Software Services Pvt. Ltd.
Cover Design: Kristin E. Parker
Rights & Media Specialist: Merideth Tumasz
Media Development Editor: Shannon Sheehan
Cover Image: Clockwise from top © Nikhil Gangavane/Dreamstime.com;
   © fenkieandreas/Shutterstock; © smereka/ShutterStock, Inc.
Printing and Binding: Edwards Brothers Malloy
Cover Printing: Edwards Brothers Malloy

Library of Congress Cataloging-in-Publication Data
Names: Riegelman, Richard K., author. | Kirkwood, Brenda, author. |
   Supplement to (expression): Riegelman, Richard K. Public health 101. 2nd ed.
Title: One Health : from AIDS to Zika / Richard Riegelman, Brenda Kirkwood.
Description: Burlington, Massachusetts : Jones & Bartlett Learning, [2018] |
   Includes bibliographical references.
Identifiers: LCCN 2016033364 | ISBN 9781284136746 (pbk.)
Subjects: | MESH: One Health (Initiative). | Virus Diseases—etiology |
   Zoonoses
Classification: LCC RC114.5 | NLM WC 500 | DDC 362.1969/1—dc23
LC record available at https://lccn.loc.gov/2016033364

6048

Printed in the United States of America
20 19 18 17 16   10 9 8 7 6 5 4 3 2 1

TABLE OF CONTENTS

II. ECOSYSTEM HEALTH/PHYSICAL ENVIRONMENT

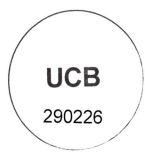

LEARNING OBJECTIVES

Students completing this material will be able to:

- Explain the components of the One Health educational framework
- Discuss the history and need for the One Health Initiative
- Illustrate microbiological influences on health and disease
- Analyze how ecosystem changes affect human health
- Discuss human–animal interactions and their positive and negative impacts on health and disease
- Describe global efforts to recognize and control pandemic disease

One Health focuses on the connections among human, animal, and ecosystem health, as illustrated in **Figure 1**.

One Health contends that human health is dependent on animal health and the health of the ecosystem. "We're all in it together" is no longer just about the human race; it is about the health of all living things.

We examine the three components of the One Health educational framework as developed by the One Health Interprofessional Education Working Group,[a] which is made up of representatives of medicine, nursing, pharmacy, and veterinary medicine, as well as public health.[1] These components include:

- Microbiological influences on health and disease
- Ecosystem health/physical environment
- Human–animal interaction

Before we examine each of these components, let us take a look at where the One Health movement comes from and why a new movement is needed.

WHERE DID THE CONCEPT OF ONE HEALTH ORIGINATE?

The One Health concept builds on the traditional means of controlling zoonotic disease. Zoonotic diseases are diseases that can be passed between animals and humans. Control and prevention of infectious diseases, including those shared by animals and humans, was one of the great public health achievements of the first half of the 20th century in the United States

---

[a] The One Health Interprofessional Education Working Group was convened by the Association of American Veterinary Medical Colleges with the collaboration of the Healthy People Curriculum Taskforce of the Association for Prevention Teaching and Research.

Figure 1 One Health: Human Health, Animal Health, and Ecosystem Health

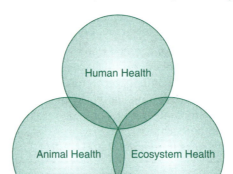

The relationships among human health, animal health, and ecosystem health are central to One Health.

and many developed countries. Nevertheless, throughout the world, much remains to be done on this front.

The following three examples demonstrate the successes and continuing challenges of control of zoonotic diseases.

Anthrax

Anthrax is an ancient disease of grazing animals. According to the Centers for Disease Control and Prevention (CDC), during Moses's time, anthrax may have been the cause of the "fifth plague," which affected horses, cattle, sheep, camels, and oxen. Anthrax is a spore-producing bacterium that can be transmitted from animals to humans through skin contact with infected animals, consumption of their food by-products, or airborne exposure. Anthrax played an important role in the 19th-century bacteriology revolution. Robert Koch used anthrax to develop Koch's Postulates—his requirements to establish the cause of a bacterial disease. Although Louis Pasteur developed the first vaccine for anthrax in the late 1800s, widespread animal vaccination did not become available until the late 1930s. After its introduction in the 1940s, penicillin quickly became the human treatment of choice. In turn, anthrax became extremely rare in the United States in the last half of the 20th century. However, anthrax again took center stage in 2001 as an agent of bioterrorism soon after the terrorist attacks on September 11 of that year. Letters laced with anthrax killed 5 Americans and sickened

17 in what became known as "Amerithrax," the worst biological attacks in U.S. history.[2]

Rabies

Since ancient times it has been known that dogs and, to a lesser degree, cats are the main source of human rabies. Control of stray dogs and cats and quarantine or euthanasia of suspicious animals have been practiced for many years and are still a mainstay of control of rabies. It was not until the development of a vaccine, however, that human rabies came under control. Louis Pasteur is credited with developing the first human rabies vaccine, but it was not until the 1920s that a vaccine for domestic pets became widely available and was largely successful in controlling rabies at least in developed countries. Rabies remains widespread in wildlife and is the major source of human exposure in most developed countries. Human rabies may result from direct wildlife exposure or via exposure of domestic or stray animals including small mammals.[3]

Bovine Tuberculosis

Tuberculosis (TB) was named after the "tubercles" or enlarged lymph nodes in cattle that are characteristic of bovine TB. During the early years of the 20th century, bovine TB is believed to have been responsible for more losses among farm animals, especially cows, than any other infectious disease. *Mycobacterium bovis,* the causative organism, is usually transmitted to humans by consuming raw cow's milk that is infected with the bacterium and can lead to the development of active TB in humans. During the early 20th century, bovine TB was controlled or eliminated in the United States and in most other developed countries through pasteurization of milk and the testing and "culling" or slaughter of animals with the disease. In most developed countries today, bovine TB is rare in farm animals and in humans. In areas without effective control of bovine TB, it remains a major cause of human TB.[4]

Box 1 provides a brief history of the efforts to control zoonotic diseases, beginning with Rudolph Virchow, who coined the term "zoonotic disease."

The control of zoonotic diseases was part of wider efforts to control infectious diseases in the first half of the 20th century. The overall impact of these efforts is reflected in life expectancy at birth, or the average number of years a newborn can be expected to live based on the conditions in a

---

BOX 1 CONTROL OF ZOONOTIC DISEASES

The history of the One Health concept can be traced to Rudolph Virchow, a 19th-century German pathologist and public health leader who coined the term "zoonotic disease." We now know that zoonotic diseases can be caused by viruses, bacteria, parasites, and fungi.

One of Virchow's important contributions was establishing the roundworm *Trichinella* as the cause of trichinosis, a painful and potentially fatal disease in humans that affects the muscles. Trichinosis is caused by eating raw or undercooked pork as well as through consumption of many wildlife species that contain the roundworm larvae.

Virchow's public health activism included convincing the German people that "Rawfleisch" (lightly smoke-cured ham), a national food specialty, and other undercooked pork dishes were the principal cause of trichinosis.[5] According to the National Institutes of Health (NIH) website, Virchow was opposed to Otto von Bismarck's military budget, "which angered Bismarck sufficiently to challenge Virchow to a duel. Virchow, being entitled to choose the weapons, chose 2 pork sausages: a cooked sausage for himself and an uncooked one, loaded with *Trichinella* larvae, for Bismarck. Bismarck, the Iron Chancellor, declined the proposition as too risky."[6]

Virchow's understanding of the relationship between animal and human disease led him to promote an approach bridging the divide between human medicine and veterinary medicine. These early insights into the relationship between human and animal health were brought to the United States by William Osler, an early advocate of understanding the connections between human and animal health. Virchow's aphorism "between animal and human medicine there are no dividing lines—nor should there be" came to symbolize the efforts to control zoonotic diseases.[7]

---

particular year. Life expectancy in the United States in 1900 was 47 years; in 1950, it was 68 years. A large proportion of this improvement was due to control of infectious diseases. In 1900, the number of deaths due to infectious diseases per 100,000 population was about 500. This number declined to approximately 30 per 100,000 by 1950.[8]

WHY IS A NEW MOVEMENT NEEDED?

By the 1960s and 1970s, the medical and public health communities often felt that victory was in sight in the battle against infectious diseases. Antibiotics were curing most bacterial diseases, including tuberculosis; vaccines were controlling many viral disease outbreaks; and smallpox eradication was on the horizon. Malaria and other mosquito-borne disease had been reduced by widespread mosquito control, often through use of DDT and other pesticides. There was so much confidence even among scientists that success would continue that you could count on one hand the number of yearly scientific papers that dealt with new or emerging infectious diseases.[9]

All that began to change in the 1980s with the emergence of HIV/AIDS and the recognition that it likely had its origins in the African tropical forests. Mosquito-borne diseases, including dengue fever, West Nile virus, Chikungunya, and most recently Zika virus, began a relentless expansion. In addition, new life-threatening diseases—most notably severe acute respiratory syndrome (SARS)—emerged and rapidly spread from person to person, posing the threat of international epidemics and disrupting the rapid growth of global trade as well as international travel.[10]

In the 21st century it has become evident that environmental change, population growth, and economic disparities have accelerated the pace of spread of existing diseases. A new form of cholera more resistant to control has developed in areas of poverty and poor sanitation. Existing vector-borne diseases, especially those transmitted by mosquitos, are extending their territory due to climate change. Intensive "industrial" production of animals for human food has made more likely an influenza A pandemic due to mutations taking place in swine feedlots. Extensive use of antibiotics for animal growth and disease prevention has contributed to development of antibiotic-resistant bacteria. It is now apparent that we need to take a new look at the relationships among humans, animals, and the ecosystem and better understand their connections. That is what One Health is all about.

WHAT IS THE ONE HEALTH INITIATIVE?

The One Health Initiative has been a response to these increasing threats. Developed initially by the veterinary medicine community, it has been widely accepted by national and international organizations.[b] The One Health Initiative defines One Health as "the collaborative effort of multiple health science professions, together with their related disciplines and institutions—working locally, nationally, and globally—to attain optimal health for people, domestic animals, wildlife, plants, and our environment."[11]

---

[b] The organizations include CDC, the World Health Organization (WHO), the World Organization for Animal Health (OIE), the European Union, and the World Bank.

One Health is designed to serve as an umbrella organization under which collaboration is facilitated between the full range of disciplines and professions that connect human health, animal health, and health of the ecosystem, as illustrated in the One Health "umbrella" depicted in **Figure 2**. Note that public health and population health are in the center under the umbrella but a wide range of other disciplines and professions are needed to accomplish the goals of One Health. Public health can play a key role in helping bring the ideas and talents that are needed to address both immediate and future issues related to interactions among human, animal, and ecosystem health.

We examine the One Health Initiative mostly from the perspective of human health. Ideally, however, these benefits flow both ways. Animals may also benefit from control of zoonotic diseases and from the human–animal bond. In addition, reducing the rate of human-mediated species loss and artificial introduction of non-native species may help sustain ecosystems.

Figure 2 The One Health Umbrella Indicating the Need for Broad Collaboration to Achieve the Goals of One Health

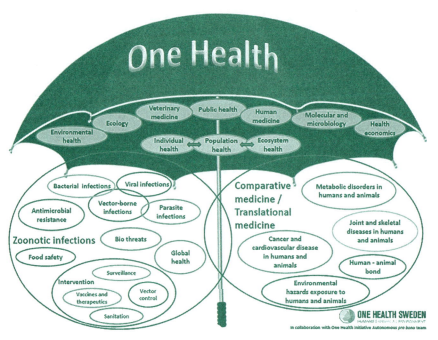

The One Health Initiative aims to encourage collaboration between professions and disciplines under the One Health umbrella.

Reproduced from One Health Initiative. About the One Health Initiative. http://www .onehealthinitiative.com/about.php. Accessed June 27, 2016.

To understand One Health, it is important to define a number of key terms. These are included in **Box 2**.

We are now ready to examine each of the three components of One Health, starting with the microbiological influences on health and disease.

BOX 2 KEY ONE HEALTH TERMS

The following definitions reflect the use of these terms in *One Health: From AIDS to Zika*.

Animal reservoirs Human pathogens often have animal reservoirs that may serve as the source of human infection because of the ability of the organism to multiply or "amplify" in the animal with or without producing symptoms in the host. Reservoirs of human pathogens also include plants and soil.

Case-fatality rate The chances of dying from a condition once it is diagnosed.

Communicable disease A subset of infectious diseases. An infectious disease that can be transmitted from a reservoir to a susceptible human or animal host. Often used for diseases that can be transmitted person to person.

Emerging infectious diseases According to the World Health Organization (WHO), emerging infectious diseases are infectious diseases that have appeared in a population for the first time or that may have existed previously but are reemerging—that is, rapidly increasing in incidence or geographic range.

Endemic A term used when a disease is present or develops in a population or community but at a relatively low and stable rate.

Epidemic A term used when new disease or other health-related event has increased in a defined geographic area clearly in excess of the expected incidence rate, or rate of new cases. Often used to imply the rapid spread of a communicable disease.

Exotic pets This term has no firm definition; it can refer to any native or non-native wildlife kept in human households, including domestic reptiles and amphibians. Small domestic mammals may or may not be classified as exotic pets.

Infectious disease An illness resulting from the presence of a pathogenic biological agent in a host human or animal. The pathogen may or may not be communicable—that is, able to be transmitted to other humans or animals.

Microbiological A term describing pathological as well as beneficial biological agents that cannot be seen with the naked eye, including bacteria, viruses, parasites, protozoa, fungi, and prions.

Pandemic An epidemic occurring worldwide or over a wide area, often crossing international boundaries and affecting a large number of humans.

(continues)

> **BOX 2** KEY ONE HEALTH TERMS (*continued*)
>
> **Pathogen** Any biological agent that causes disease or illness to a host human or animal.
>
> **RNA virus** A virus in which the genetic material is RNA as opposed to DNA. The RNA may be either double or single stranded.
>
> **Spillover** Crossing of a pathogen from one species to another species. Often used to imply that a pathogen has been transmitted to humans without having the ability, at least initially, to be transmitted from person to person.
>
> **Transmission** Any mechanism by which a communicable disease is spread from or to a human or animal.
>
> **Vector** An animal, most often a mosquito, that plays a role in the transmission of disease from animals to humans or from humans to humans. The pathogen may or may not reproduce within the vector.
>
> **Zoonotic disease** A human disease that under natural conditions can be transmitted from vertebrate animals to humans.

I. MICROBIOLOGICAL INFLUENCES ON HEALTH AND DISEASE

WHAT ARE THE MOST IMPORTANT MICROBIOLOGICAL THREATS TO THE PUBLIC'S HEALTH?

In our discussion of zoonotic diseases, we have seen that both bacteria (anthrax and bovine tuberculosis) and viruses (rabies) can produce serious human diseases. A wide range of microbiological entities can produce human disease, including DNA and RNA viruses, bacteria, parasites, protozoa, and fungi, as well as prions, which are a disease-causing form of a normal brain protein. Whole textbooks would be required to discuss all of these agents. However, in terms of their threats of causing human epidemics and pandemics, one category—RNA viruses—is of greatest importance as regards One Health. Therefore, we focus our discussion of the microbiological influences on health and disease on RNA viruses.

Many of the most serious microbiological threats to the public's health are due to RNA viruses. There are currently approximately 200 species of RNA viruses that can infect humans, and more species are being added each year. This represents only a small fraction of the RNA viruses that exist in nature, so there is an abundance of RNA viruses that have the potential to mutate so that they can infect humans.

RNA viruses, as opposed to DNA viruses, are far more likely to produce mutations during their frequent replications because they do not have the same protective mechanism against copying or coding errors. This high rate of mutation in RNA viruses is believed to enhance their ability to cross species lines and, once established in a new species, to continue to mutate. RNA viruses often have multiple animal species as hosts and are believed to easily cross species lines, creating new host species, including human beings. Crossing of RNA viruses between similar species such as nonhuman primates and humans is believed to be more likely than crossing between less closely related species.[12]

RNA viruses that have crossed the species line and included humans in their list of hosts often do not immediately or inevitably cause severe disease or produce epidemics. Most of the recently recognized epidemic diseases caused by RNA viruses existed in humans for years, decades, or even longer before they became epidemic diseases. Often, human populations exposed to RNA viruses as well as other pathogens gain immunity and do not experience frequent or severe illnesses. However, when previously unexposed populations encounter the same pathogen, they may experience severe or epidemic disease. We are just beginning to understand why one RNA virus causes epidemic or even pandemic disease, whereas another accommodates to human beings without producing disease.

WHAT MIGHT BE CALLED THE "TOP 10" RNA VIRUSES CAUSING EMERGING INFECTIOUS DISEASES?

We now take a look at what we call the "top 10" emerging RNA viruses. These have been chosen not just for their frequency of occurrence, but also for the impact they have had and the lessons they can teach. Together they reflect the spectrum of human emerging infections caused by RNA viruses. These top 10 infections are:

- Acquired immunodeficiency syndrome (AIDS)/human immunodeficiency virus (HIV)
- Chikungunya
- Dengue
- Ebola
- Hantavirus
- Influenza A
- Middle Eastern respiratory syndrome (MERS)

- Severe acute respiratory syndrome (SARS)
- West Nile virus
- Zika

Wolfe and his colleagues have defined five stages of progression of emerging infectious disease that culminate in stage 5—that is, exclusive person-to-person transmission.[13] **Box 3** discusses these stages, which are applicable to RNA viruses as well as other emerging infectious diseases.

BOX 3 STAGES OF EMERGING INFECTIOUS DISEASES AND TOP 10 RNA VIRUSES

Let us see what is meant by each stage and indicate which of our top 10 RNA viruses are currently in each stage.

Stage 1. A microbe that is present in animals and has not been detected in humans under natural conditions. This is currently the case with many RNA viruses.

Stage 2. A pathogen with an animal reservoir that, under natural conditions, has been transmitted from animals to humans ("primary infection") but has not been transmitted directly from human to human ("secondary infection"). Example: Hantavirus.

Stage 2 also includes RNA viruses that use mosquitos to assist in their transmission from animals to humans, rather than being transmitted from person to person. Example: West Nile virus.

Stage 3. Animal pathogens that can undergo only a few cycles of secondary transmission between humans, in which there are occasional human outbreaks, even severe ones, but they can be controlled or at least temporarily die out on their own. Example: MERS.

Stage 4. A pathogen that exists in animals, and that has a natural cycle of infecting humans by primary transmission from the animal host, followed by spread primarily by person-to-person contact. Stage 4 includes a range of diseases, from ones primarily transmitted among animal species to ones primarily transmitted human to human. Examples: Influenza A, SARS, and Ebola. Stage 4 also includes infections that have primary transmission between humans through a vector such as mosquitos. Examples: Dengue fever, Chikungunya, and Zika.

Stage 5. A pathogen, without an animal reservoir, that is currently exclusively transmitted from person to person without the involvement of animal hosts or intermediate transmission via vectors. Example: AIDS/HIV.

There is no inevitable progression from stage 1 to stage 5. Most RNA viruses and other pathogens do not progress to stage 5.

WHAT IS IMPORTANT TO KNOW ABOUT EACH OF OUR TOP 10 RNA VIRUSES?

The top 10 RNA viruses reflect the range of challenges that the world confronts from emerging infections. Let us briefly review key points to know about each of the top 10 RNA viruses in alphabetical order from AIDS to Zika.

Acquired Immunodeficiency Syndrome and Human Immunodeficiency Virus

The human immunodeficiency virus, an RNA virus, is the cause of acquired immunodeficiency syndrome and is usually referred to as HIV/AIDS. Nearly 40 million people have died from the AIDS epidemic. The virus is capable of evading the human immune system and killing CD4 cells, which are central to the body's defenses. This allows the development of a wide array of potentially fatal "opportunistic infections," including tuberculosis.

Despite the fact that human immunodeficiency virus, as the name implies, is currently exclusively transmitted from person to person, recent evidence strongly supports its origin in nonhuman primates in Africa. Genetic evidence strongly implies that it was introduced into the human population in the late 1950s or perhaps multiple times over previous decades. It was not until the early 1980s that it was recognized as an emerging infectious disease. By that time, it had evolved through the five stages to exclusive human-to-human transmission, most likely by ongoing mutation. As an RNA virus, HIV continues to mutate in a process that may be accelerated by the use of or misuse of antiretroviral drugs.

HIV/AIDS illustrates the fact that an emerging disease can spill over or cross over from nonhuman primate species and may exist for many years in the human population without spreading rapidly. Continued mutations and/or the right conditions or exposures may convert a rare human infection into a rapidly spreading emerging infectious disease. HIV also illustrates the full range of determinants of disease, including the social, cultural, and economic factors affecting the spread of disease—from sexual and breast-feeding practices to use of needles to access to state-of-the-art health care.

HIV/AIDS also illustrates the potential to control communicable disease through prevention, early and rapid diagnosis, treatment of those persons with the infection, and reduction of transmission from mother to child as well as through sexual exposure, shared needle use, and blood transfusions. Research on HIV/AIDS has produced much greater understanding of the action of viruses and the potential for control of disease. Drug treatments are now allowing a large percentage of those individuals with HIV to live with the disease. However, the search for a vaccine has been exceedingly complicated and frustrating in this disease because it is caused by an RNA virus, which has demonstrated its ability to continuously mutate and to successfully evade human immune defenses.[14]

Chikungunya

Chikungunya is a classic example of an emerging infectious disease. Until the 1950s, it most likely existed only in nonhuman primates and forest-dwelling mosquitos. In the 1950s, it was first detected in humans in sub-Saharan Africa. The name Chikungunya comes from African words meaning "to become contorted" or "to walk bent over," reflecting the severe joint pain this disease produces and the efforts of patients to find a comfortable position.

The disease rapidly became established not only in Africa but also in Asia, where it was transmitted by the *Aedes aegypti* mosquito, a dawn- and dusk-biting mosquito common in tropical regions. In 2004, a mutation of Chikungunya virus was documented that allowed spread of infection with a smaller amount of the virus during mosquito feeding. This in turn allowed another mosquito species, *Aedes albopictus* (commonly called the Asian tiger mosquito), to transmit the disease.

The Asian tiger mosquito is a daytime feeder and far more aggressive in its efforts to bite and feed on humans. As its name implies, until recently it was found exclusively in Asia. Increased global trade has brought the mosquito to the United States, where it now has established itself in the southern and mid-Atlantic states. Currently, it is extending west and north because, unlike *Aedes aegypti*, it is able to withstand colder winter temperatures.

The combination of the right mutation and the right mosquito most likely led to the major outbreaks of Chikungunya in the Caribbean that in recent years have infected millions of people. Transmission has been documented in Florida. With the Asian tiger mosquito already present in much of the United States, at least sporadic cases of locally transmitted Chikungunya may not be far behind.

Fortunately, Chikungunya rarely causes death in most healthy individuals. However, in the elderly, immunosuppressed persons, and infants born to actively infected mothers, it can pose a risk of severe disease and even death. Mosquito control efforts and use of mosquito repellant are currently the only recommended preventive measures.[15]

Dengue

Dengue is an example of a long-standing human disease that has increased in frequency and expanded into new territory in recent years. Known in the United States since colonial times, dengue is transmitted by the *Aedes aegypti* mosquito.

Dengue is usually a relatively mild disease, but severe disease—known as dengue hemorrhagic fever—can occur. The CDC describes dengue hemorrhagic fever (DHF) as follows: "A fever that lasts from 2 to 7 days ... When the fever declines, symptoms including persistent vomiting, severe abdominal pain, and difficulty breathing, may develop. This marks the beginning of a 24- to 48-hour period when the smallest blood vessels (capillaries) become excessively permeable ('leaky'), allowing the fluid component to escape from the blood vessels into the peritoneum (causing ascites) and pleural cavity (leading to pleural effusions). This may lead to failure of the circulatory system and shock," and possibly death without prompt, appropriate treatment.[16(para5)]

Worldwide, an estimated 500,000 people with severe dengue require hospitalization each year, a large proportion of whom are children. Approximately 2.5% of those affected die. In 2015, 2.35 million cases of dengue were reported in the Americas alone.

Before 1970, only 9 countries had experienced severe dengue epidemics. The disease is now endemic in more than 100 countries that are home to approximately half the world's population, including countries in Africa, the Americas, the eastern Mediterranean, Southeast Asia, and the Western Pacific including Hawaii, where repeated outbreaks have occurred. The World Health Organization (WHO) reports that dengue incidence has increased 30-fold since the 1970s, when extensive use of pesticides for mosquito control was curtailed due to growing resistance and environmental destruction.

A dengue vaccine that has shown efficacy in randomized controlled trials among individuals 9 years and older has been developed. The vaccine requires three doses over a 12-month period. WHO's Strategic Advisory Group of Experts (SAGE) has recommended use of the vaccine only for populations at very high risk and only when combined with a comprehensive program of prevention and treatment. The vaccine holds promise of having a major impact, especially against severe dengue, but dengue shows no signs of going away.[17,18]

Ebola

Ebola, another RNA virus, was first identified in 1976 near the Ebola River in what is now the Democratic Republic of the Congo. Since then, more than 25 outbreaks including person-to-person transmission have appeared sporadically in Africa. Ebola, which causes Ebola hemorrhagic fever, is a tragic disease in which patients experience internal and external bleeding and damage to almost every organ before succumbing to the infection. As the disease progresses, the virus is contained in the blood and body fluids (including but not limited to urine, saliva, sweat, feces, vomit, breast milk, and semen), making it potentially contagious through close contact as well as through needlesticks. For those who recover, the virus can remain in their bodies for long periods of time. It is not known whether those who have recovered continue to have the potential to transmit the disease.

The natural reservoir host of Ebola virus remains unconfirmed. However, researchers believe that bats are the most likely reservoir species and the initial source of the infection in human and nonhuman primates. Nonhuman primates are susceptible to Ebola and have died in large numbers from this disease. Four different species of Ebola can cause disease, so it is possible for individuals to contract Ebola more than once.

Previous Ebola outbreaks occurred in sparsely populated rural areas where the potential to perpetuate the epidemic by person-to-person transmission was limited. The 2014–2016 epidemic of Ebola was different because it spread rapidly across three West African countries, including their densely populated capital cities, causing nearly 30,000 cases and 11,000 deaths. The fatalities included more than 500 deaths among healthcare workers who experienced close personal contact with those infected with the disease. There were more than 10 times as many cases of Ebola in the 2014–2016 epidemic as in all the previous outbreaks combined.

Cultural factors increased the spread of the disease. Family and friends in affected areas often had close contact with the terminally ill as well as the bodies of the deceased, increasing the spread of Ebola. Providing safe and dignified burials for Ebola victims has become an important method for controlling the epidemic.

Fear of the disease spread even faster than the disease itself when individuals infected with Ebola, especially those still without symptoms, returned to Europe and North America. Person-to-person transmission occurred among close contacts and healthcare workers once symptoms of Ebola appeared. Specialized units set up to handle Ebola were needed. A coordinated international effort helped control the epidemic in Africa, including the use of U.S. military personnel as well as public health workers from the CDC and international organizations.

The lingering effects of the latest Ebola epidemic include the potential to create panic around the world due to the dramatic and devastating nature of the disease. Efforts to prepare for and organize rapid responses to future localized epidemics of Ebola and other emerging diseases will be a legacy of the Ebola epidemic, as we discuss in the final section on putting One Health into practice.[19]

Hantavirus

Though a rare disease in humans that cannot be transmitted from person to person, hantavirus is included as one of our top 10 RNA diseases because it reflects how humans can develop disease through routine exposures to nature and how disease can be prevented. Hantavirus is carried by mice and other rodents in some parts of the United States, especially the Southwest and West.

Although first isolated in Korea in 1976, hantaviruses were not recognized in the United States until 1993, when an outbreak with a high case-fatality rate occurred among Navajos. At that time, the disease was given the name Sin Nombre, Spanish for "nameless." The Sin Nombre hantavirus, among the first to be identified by the then new polymerase chain reaction (PCR) technology, caused severe and often fatal lung disease among previously healthy individuals. Lung disease had not previously been a known complication of hantavirus infection. The disease might have been endemic in the area for centuries because Navajo tradition recognized similar disease and linked it to mice.

Transmission usually occurs when humans breathe the virus contained in rodent urine or feces that has become airborne or aerosolized. Weeks later, a small percentage of those exposed to hantavirus develop respiratory infection, which initially is indistinguishable from the common cold but can rapidly progress to respiratory failure. This condition, called hantavirus pulmonary syndrome, has a case-fatality rate of more than one-third.

The most widely publicized hantavirus outbreak in recent years occurred in Yosemite National Park. A large number of cases and three deaths occurred there in 2012 in newly constructed cabins that were found to harbor rodent nests in their insulation.

The CDC reports that hantavirus infection is most likely to occur when opening and cleaning previously unused spaces, when cleaning homes in areas with rodent droppings, in construction and pest control (especially in crawl spaces), and among campers and hikers (especially in trail shelters).[20,21]

Hantavirus illustrates how new or previously unrecognized diseases from human–animal contact can appear in very unexpected places, including the most natural and beautiful settings in the United States.

Influenza A

Influenza A has been an ongoing annual threat to health for many years, as evidenced by the 1918–1919 pandemic. The worst pandemic of the 20th century, it killed approximately 50 million people, many of whom were previously young and healthy. Influenza A remains a disease that affects humans by person-to-person respiratory transmission. Wild birds and pigs or swine serve as reservoirs and provide opportunities for the emergence of new strains. The mixing of the different subtypes of the virus is believed to allow genetic changes, which may result in new subtypes capable of human-to-human respiratory transmission.

Mutations in the influenza A virus are a continuous phenomenon capable of producing new subtypes on a regular basis. Each year the CDC attempts to predict the dominant strains in time to allow preparation of protective vaccines. In some—but not all—years, this effort has been successful, leading to a reduction in the number of cases and the number of deaths. Death rates vary greatly from year to year, but on average nearly 30,000 individuals die during each flu season from influenza A in the United States, a disproportionate number of whom are very young, very old, or chronically ill.

When a major change in the influenza A virus occurs, previous immunity does not provide protection from the disease. In this situation the entire population may be susceptible, potentially leading to a worldwide pandemic. In 2009–2010, an influenza A pandemic occurred because of a new strain that is believed to have been transmitted to humans from swine in Mexico and rapidly spread to the United States and beyond. Fortunately, the 2009 pandemic did not result in a high case-fatality rate, but the same might not be true in future pandemics.

Progress in rapidly producing and distributing vaccines holds promise in minimizing the national and global impact of influenza A. In the United States, efforts to make current vaccines widely available and affordable through pharmacies and other retail outlets have already had an impact on the occurrence and mortality from this ongoing, continuously reemerging disease.[22]

Middle Eastern Respiratory Syndrome

Middle Eastern respiratory syndrome (MERS) is a newly recognized coronavirus (CoV) related to SARS. Like SARS, MERS affects the respiratory system. Most patients with MERS develop severe acute respiratory illness with symptoms of fever, cough, and shortness of breath. Three to four of every 10 patients reported with MERS have died.

The CDC reports that the first cases of the disease were recognized in Saudi Arabia in 2012. Approximately 2,000 people have developed the disease, and about 25% have died. So far, all cases of MERS around the world, including those in the United States, have been linked to travel to or residence in countries in and near the Arabian Peninsula. MERS CoV has spread from ill people to others through close contact, such as caring for or living with an infected person. MERS patients have ranged in age from younger than 1 to 99 years old. Most of the people who have died have had underlying medical conditions that weakened their immune responses.

MERS CoV has been found in camels, and some MERS patients have reported contact with camels. The WHO suggests general precautions for anyone visiting farms, markets, barns, or other places in affected countries where animals are present. Travelers should practice general hygiene measures, including regular hand washing before and after touching animals, and avoid contact with sick animals. Travelers should also avoid consumption of raw or undercooked animal products, especially camel meat.

Avoiding drinking raw camel's milk is also strongly recommended by WHO. Camel traders have been accused of facilitating entry of MERS into the human population through drinking such milk. One attention-getting WHO recommendation is to avoid the practice of drinking camel urine to avoid or cure disease—a practice found in parts of the Arabian Peninsula. Thus, once again, cultural practices have been found to play a role in the development of emerging infectious disease.

MERS has not been shown to cause disease by person-to-person transmission beyond those in close contact with a sick MERS patient. However, the recent outbreak in South Korea shows the potential for widespread dissemination of MERS. In the summer of 2015, an outbreak of MERS occurred among nearly 100 people in South Korea, approximately 25% of whom died. The outbreak was traced to a single patient with MERS returning from the Arabian Peninsula.[23,24]

Severe Acute Respiratory Syndrome

We now know that the 2003 outbreak of severe acute respiratory syndrome (SARS) that nearly shut down international air travel and threatened international trade began somewhere in Guangdong Province in southwestern China. Guangdong Province, which is home to 79 million people, is less than 100 miles up the Pearl River from Hong Kong, where the first cases of SARS were identified. In this area of China, civet cats—which are actually not cats, but a relative of the mongoose—are eaten as a delicacy in the winter. They are hunted, raised on farms, and sold in markets. The SARS coronavirus has been traced to a mutation of the RNA coronavirus carried by civet cats, which shed large numbers of the virus in their feces.

It is now well established that once the disease took hold in humans, it could be transmitted by airborne aerosol droplets. SARS was able to quickly spread to 30 countries, causing 8,000 cases and 800 deaths.

The documentation of a small number of "super spreaders" was shown to greatly enhance the potential for epidemic spread. Fortunately, with careful isolation and quarantine, person-to-person spread of SARS was interrupted and there have not been any recent reports of its reemergence. Despite the absence of reported human cases in recent years, given its animal reservoirs in bats and its ability to infect civet cats, a reemergence of this disease is always possible.

SARS was a wake-up call for the world about the potential for widespread death and disruption that can occur from an emerging infectious disease, most often an RNA virus. The world did respond to SARS with measures including, as we discuss later, providing the WHO with new authority and new responsibility as well as initiating the development of a worldwide network of public health institutes that are providing rapid access to technology and resources needed to address health emergencies. Finally, the international attention generated by SARS provided fertile ground for the initial development of the One Health Initiative. The successful international collaboration stimulated by SARS provides hope for our ability to address a wide range of emerging infectious diseases.[25,26]

West Nile Virus

West Nile virus was first recognized in 1937 in the West Nile region of Uganda and was soon identified in parts of the Middle East. It usually caused mild disease. In the late 1990s, it began to spread to other regions, perhaps due to a recently recognized mutation. It reached New York City in 1999 and spread throughout the continental United States over the next 5 years.

West Nile virus is often transmitted in the late summer or early fall to humans and horses by the bite of the *Culex* mosquito, better known as the common house mosquito. The *Culex* mosquito typically obtains its blood meal from birds instead of humans, but can then transmit the virus to humans when it subsequently bites humans, usually at dawn or dusk.

The American crow and other related species, which are common in most of the United States, are particularly prone to West Nile infection and produce high levels of the virus in their blood, allowing mosquitos to transmit the disease from birds to humans. Public health surveillance for West Nile virus often monitors the disease in crows and other bird species as an indication of impending disease in humans. The severity of the disease in some bird species has led to the disease becoming a conservation concern and created uncertainty about the long-term impacts of reductions in certain bird species on the function of the ecosystem.

For approximately 80% of people who are exposed to the West Nile virus, the disease does not produce symptoms. Most of the remaining 20% experience a brief period of fever and nonspecific symptoms such as headache, joint pain, and nausea. Fewer than 1% develop severe neurologic disease, which can include high fever, neck stiffness, disorientation, coma, tremors, seizures, or paralysis. There is a 10% case-fatality rate with severe disease, and other patients are left with permanent neurologic damage. Severe disease is more common among those persons older than age 60 and those individuals with diseases or treatments that impair their immunologic response. Despite the inability to transmit the disease directly from person to person, West Nile virus has been shown to be transmissible from mother to child through intrauterine exposure and breastfeeding as well as through blood transfusions and organ transplants.

There is no human vaccine that can protect against infection of West Nile virus, although a DNA vaccine is available for horses. Research on the safety and efficacy of the horse vaccine may shed light on the safety and effectiveness of this new form of vaccination for humans.[27]

Zika Virus

In 1947, researchers identified a new virus in a rhesus monkey in the Zika forest of Uganda, naming it Zika virus. The virus was soon isolated from mosquitos from the same forest, suggesting mosquito-borne transmission of this pathogen. The first human cases of Zika virus infection were identified in 1952. More than a decade later, a researcher studying Zika virus was accidently infected and developed mild disease, indicating the potential for Zika, an RNA virus, to become a human pathogen.

From the 1960s through the 1980s, the spread of Zika virus was traced to Central and West Africa as well as tropical areas of Asia. Evidence of infection was found to be widespread, but there was little evidence of symptoms or complications. When symptoms did occur, they resembled mild self-limited cases of dengue fever or Chikungunya with fever, rash, and joint pain.

The first large outbreak of human disease caused by Zika virus occurred in 2004 on the Micronesian island of Yap, where the population had no history of prior exposure to Zika virus. More than 70% of the residents were infected. Outbreaks on other Polynesian islands in 2013 and 2014 suggested for the first time that Zika virus can cross the placental barrier and infect a fetus. Later studies of these populations also identified a large increase in neurologic disease including Guillain–Barré syndrome, a rare, rapidly progressing, and potentially fatal neurologic disease.

The world learned of Zika virus in 2015, after physicians in poverty-stricken northeast Brazil reported an enormous increase in the number of new cases of microcephaly in newborns whose mothers were found to have had Zika virus infection during pregnancy. Studies soon established that Zika virus can invade the brain of a fetus and cause direct injury to the developing brain. Epidemiologic and laboratory investigations confirmed that Zika virus can cause microcephaly and other diseases of the newborn, including eye disease.

In 2015 and 2016, Zika virus spread rapidly throughout South America and Central America and the Caribbean, transmitted by *Aedes aegypti* mosquitos. Mosquito-borne transmission can be expected in the Americas, including the United States, wherever *Aedes aegypti* mosquitos thrive. In addition, sexual transmission was confirmed with the potential for transmission for extended periods after initial infection. Therefore, Zika can be acquired by more than one type of transmission—both direct person-to-person transmission and via mosquito bites.[28,29]

Much remains to be learned about the Zika virus, but it is already all too clear that it is an emerging infectious disease that illustrates how rare emerging diseases that spill over from other species can suddenly and unexpectedly emerge as epidemic and even pandemic diseases. Zika virus also indicates how much we still have to learn about how infectious diseases emerge, which types of infections they can cause, and how we can prevent, control, and treat these infections.

Our top 10 RNA viruses illustrate the diverse challenges that humans face. Social and economic factors as well as individual behavior and local cultures all play a role in determining where, when, and how many individuals will be affected by RNA viruses and other infectious diseases. We will return to the issue of what we can do to prevent and control RNA viruses, but first let us take a look at the second component of the One Health educational framework: ecosystem health/physical environment.

II. ECOSYSTEM HEALTH/PHYSICAL ENVIRONMENT

Ecosystem health and its impact on human health involve a wide range of factors that directly affect the physical world in which we live.[30] We examine how changes in the following factors can have major impacts on human health:

- Global movement of populations
- Agriculture changes and changes in food distribution
- Ecological changes in land and resource use
- Misuse of technologies that affect the ecosystem
- Climate change

In addition, we need to keep in mind key underlying mechanisms that often affect these factors. These mechanisms include poverty and social-economic conditions as well as population growth.

The factors that directly affect the ecosystem and human health can often be affected by poverty and the social and environmental conditions created by poverty. Therefore, it should not be surprising that changes in socioeconomic conditions can alter these factors for better or for worse as we illustrate in examples that follow. Because of the connection between socioeconomic factors and the health of the ecosystem, environmental health is increasingly being linked to the broader concept of social determinants of health.

Population growth also has a direct impact on ecosystem health through human presence in previously uninhabited areas as well as an indirect impact through increased demands for food and other resources that lead to potentially damaging impacts on the environment. The impacts of population growth continue in many areas of the developing world and have both subtle and not so subtle impacts on ecosystems.

HOW CAN GLOBAL MOVEMENTS OF POPULATIONS AFFECT HEALTH?

Major migrations of human populations and exposure to new diseases have been accompanied by epidemic and pandemic spread of disease. Anthony Fauci, Director of the National Institute of Allergy and Infectious Diseases (NIAID), and his colleagues have described the two-way expansion of disease caused by the exploration and conquest of the Americas as follows:

> *From the 15th through to the 19th century, a time when previously isolated continents were discovering each other and thereby exchanging microorganisms, reemergence of epidemic diseases associated with geographic spread of microbes became common. In December 1494, a new disease emerged in Italy; prostitutes from Naples soon infected soldiers from an invading French army. By July the disease was being diagnosed in mercenaries from Flanders, Gascony (southwest France), Switzerland, Italy, Spain, and elsewhere; they eventually returned home and spread it throughout Europe.*[31(p712)]

This disease was what we today call syphilis. Fauci et al. write that "strong evidence for New World exportation was eventually provided by testimony from Columbus' men and by physicians' accounts that Hispaniola natives had been affected by the disease since ancient times."[31(p713)]

Europeans also brought epidemic diseases to the Americas. The Spanish brought smallpox to the Americas in the early 1500s. As Fauci et al indicate: "Although smallpox may have first emerged in central Africa 5,000 years previously ... the disease had probably not reached the New World. Historians believe that about 3.5 million people in central Mexico died in the first year.... By the end of the century some 18.5 (74%) of the 25 million population had died, presumably largely because of smallpox and additional imported diseases. Smallpox spread southward into South America, ultimately destroying two great civilizations, the Aztec and Inca empires, facilitating Spanish conquests that greatly altered history."[31(p713),c]

Today's movement of populations dwarfs those of 500 years ago and 100 years ago. The ability to move around the globe in hours rather than days or

---

[c] According to Fauci et al., "Francisco Pizarro, who continued Spanish conquests of South America in the 1530s, is alleged to have undertaken a bioterrorist attack on native peoples using smallpox contaminated blankets. Mexico became a regional geographic reservoir for smallpox and was the source of repeated exportations until the 1940s."[31(p713)]

months has created the potential for extraordinarily rapid spread of disease, as we saw with the SARS epidemic and are now witnessing with the Zika virus. Today, large-scale movements of populations include those caused by humanitarian crises. In the not too distant future, they may be caused by climate change as well. These large-scale movements of people may complicate efforts to prevent the outbreak of a wide range of communicable diseases. The impact of population movements is likely to fall most heavily on those countries and populations with the fewest resources to effectively respond to these threats.

HOW CAN AGRICULTURAL PRACTICES AND CHANGES IN FOOD DISTRIBUTION INFLUENCE THE OCCURRENCE OF INFECTIOUS DISEASES IN HUMANS?

Zoonotic diseases such as anthrax and bovine TB have been exacerbated by agricultural changes since humans first developed agricultural practices more than 10,000 years ago. Today we are developing new ways to produce and distribute food, which pose new types of threats. The United States, which is a net exporter of food, actually imports food from more than 100 countries.

Some agricultural practices affect not only human health but also animal health and the health of the ecosystem and, therefore, have enormous potential economic impacts. The use and misuse of pesticides, for instance, has raised concerns ranging from the health effects of human exposure to the destructive impacts on pollinating bees, which are essential for food production.

An example of the impact of recent changes in agriculture is the way that livestock and poultry are raised.[32] The increased affluence in many parts of the world and the continued growth in populations have led to a demand for more animals raised for food. A "livestock revolution" began in the 1980s that focused on the rapid expansion of intensive pig and poultry production as well as the growth of milk production. This "industrial" food production system resulted in close confinement of animals that are often inbred to maximize growth. It was also accompanied by rapid expansion of the use of antibiotics designed to prevent disease and to increase animal weight. As we will see, this livestock revolution has contributed to the development of antibiotic resistance in animals and humans.

Although the livestock revolution increased production, it also increased the risk of emerging and reemerging infectious diseases. Most dramatically, it has been at the forefront of the emergence of new strains of influenza A. The 2009–2010 influenza pandemic was first recognized among industrially raised pigs in Mexico and rapidly spread to the United States and beyond. In 2015, a highly pathogenic avian influenza strain spread rapidly through industrially raised U.S. poultry. Approximately 50 million chickens, ducks, and turkeys were infected with the virus, requiring large-scale euthanasia of entire flocks. Despite the fact that this particular strain of avian flu was not transmissible to humans, avian influenza in the United States cost farmers billions of dollars and more than doubled the price of eggs in the United States despite a large-scale increase in imports.[33]

HOW CAN ECOLOGICAL CHANGES IN LAND AND RESOURCE USE AFFECT THE DEVELOPMENT OF INFECTIOUS DISEASES?

A wide range of ecological changes can increase or reduce the frequency of infectious diseases. For instance, the building of dams has been shown to increase the presence of schistosomiasis, which affects approximately 200 million, mostly poor people in the developing world. Schistosomiasis is caused by a flatworm that develops within freshwater snails that thrive in slow-moving, vegetation-heavy water bodies. Dam construction produces ideal conditions for the disease to proliferate, often affecting those who swim or wade in infected waters and spreading quite frequently to the bladder and other organs where it can produce severe disease.[34]

Lyme disease is an example closer to home. Incidence of Lyme disease, which is transmitted to humans by tick bites, has increased dramatically in the United States in the 21st century, affecting as many as 300,000 people each year. Lyme disease has been associated with increases in forest land and increased exposure to forests, especially in the eastern United States. The growth in cases of Lyme disease has also been associated with an increase in the deer population and the white-footed mice population, which serve as part of the life cycle of ticks and provide a reservoir for the bacteria that cause Lyme disease. A controversy exists about the ability to control Lyme disease though reduction in the deer population.[35]

Environmental changes may result from natural disasters such as earth-quakes, especially when they are compounded by the impacts of poverty and unsanitary living conditions. The ongoing cholera epidemic in Haiti began after the devastating earthquake of 2010. The introduction of cholera was traced to importation of this disease by United Nations (UN) troops from Nepal. More than 500,000 cases of cholera have been reported in

Haiti. Once established in the poor sanitary conditions of Haiti, cholera has remained an ongoing threat.[36]

Not all environmental changes are detrimental to health. Chagas disease, caused by a parasite, is transmitted to animals and people by insect vectors and can cause chronic heart and intestinal diseases. More than 8 million cases attributed to local disease transmission are estimated to be found in the Americas, mainly in rural areas of Mexico, Central America, and South America, where poverty is widespread. The bugs are found in houses made from materials such as mud, adobe, straw, and palm thatch. Improvements in living standards and changes in the environment in which people live, especially better housing, are contributing to the reduction in new cases of Chagas disease.[37]

HOW CAN MISUSE OF TECHNOLOGIES AFFECT THE ECOSYSTEM AND HUMAN HEALTH?

A growing list of technologies can have intended or unintended impacts on the ecosystem. A now classic example is the hole in the atmospheric ozone layer, which is suspected to have led to greatly increased rates of melanoma and other skin cancers. The hole in the ozone resulted largely from the use of chlorofluorocarbons (CFCs)—chemicals that were formerly found in aerosol spray cans and refrigerants. The Montreal Protocol, an international agreement signed by nearly 200 countries in the late 1980s, has been largely successful in eliminating the use of CFCs and gradually restoring the ozone layer. It serves as an important precedent illustrating the potential for global cooperation to control the environmental impacts of technology on the environment.[38]

Today a major technological concern is the relationship between antibiotic use and changes in the ecosystem leading to human disease arising from antibiotic-resistant bacteria. When penicillin was first introduced in clinical practice during World War II, it had dramatic impacts on a range of infectious diseases, from pneumococcal pneumonia to *Neisseria gonorrhoeae* infection to staphylococcal wound infections. No randomized controlled trials were needed to demonstrate its efficacy or effectiveness compared to previous treatments. In short order, however, higher dosages of penicillin were required. By the early 1950s, penicillin stopped working altogether for a growing number of infections.

In the 1950s, new classes of antibiotics were developed that headed off a crisis. However, it was already apparent that bacteria had the ability to develop resistance to antibiotics using a range of mechanisms. The more aggressively antibiotics were used, the more common resistance became, especially in hospitals where antibiotics had literally become standard operating procedure.

By the early years of this century, the problem of antibiotic resistance returned with a vengeance. Today, the CDC estimates that there are more than 2 million infections per year involving antibiotic-resistant bacteria and more than 20,000 deaths from this cause each year.[39]

Misuse of antibiotics in human medicine has been common. In addition to the use of antibiotics to treat specific human bacterial infection, it became common clinical practice to try antibiotics as a first-line approach when the cause of the problem was not clear or was most likely due to a virus.

In addition, it was found that antibiotics could modestly increase the growth rate of many animals raised for food. Widespread use of low-dose antibiotics in farm animals for prevention of disease allowed the development of feedlots. As we have discussed, whole industries are now devoted to raising animals together in close quarters.

By the late 20th century, animal use of antibiotics far exceeded human use. These antibiotics often ended up in public water systems when the runoff from feedlots contaminated streams and groundwater. This phenomenon has been called a "double hit" to the ecosystem: We get antibiotics in our food and drinking water, both of which promote bacterial resistance. This situation is now rapidly changing. Today, routine feeding of medically important antibiotics for growth promotion is banned or will soon be banned in much of the developed world, including the United States.[40]

Considerable attention is now being focused on what can be done to reduce antibiotic resistance. Judicious use of therapeutic antimicrobials is an integral part of human and veterinary medical practice. It is key to maximizing therapeutic effectiveness and minimizing selection of all kinds of resistant microorganisms, not just bacteria. New drugs, greater use of vaccines, increased use of hand washing, more judicious use of antibiotics in humans and animals, along with reduced use of antibiotics in food-producing animals for growth and disease prevention are all being recommended as part of a concerted effort to address antibiotic resistance.[41] In the not too distant future, we hope to look back to the time when we turned the corner on misuse of antibiotics and other antimicrobials.

Last but not least, let us take a look at the controversial but increasingly important issue of climate change.

HOW CAN CLIMATE CHANGE AFFECT HUMAN HEALTH?

The Impacts of Climate Change on Human Health in the United States: A Scientific Assessment (Health Impacts of Climate Change Report) was published in 2016 as part of the President's Climate Action Plan.[42] It assessed the scientific evidence for a wide range of potential climate impacts on human health over the next 15 to 35 years, including heat-related deaths and disasters as well as the impacts on air quality, water quality, and distribution of vectors and vector-borne disease. These impacts affect human health through various pathways, depicted in **Figure 3**. The report used the framework in Figure 3 to analyze the impacts of climate change.

The Health Impacts of Climate Change Report focused on human health even though climate change is expected to have major impacts on animal health and environmental health. The report included a wide range of examples of potential impacts on health, as described in **Table 1**. It also developed key findings and categorized them according to the confidence in the finding based on the strength of the evidence, ranging from very high to low. In addition, the report indicated the likelihood of occurrence, ranging from very likely to very unlikely.[d]

Among the report's key findings that scored very high or high on confidence and also very likely or likely were the impacts described in the following subsections.

Exacerbated Ozone Health Impacts

Key Finding: "Climate change will make it harder for any given regulatory approach to reduce ground-level ozone pollution in the future as meteorological conditions become increasingly conducive to forming ozone over most of the United States *[Likely, High Confidence]*. Unless offset by additional emissions reductions of ozone precursors, these climate-driven increases in ozone will cause premature deaths, hospital visits, lost school days, and acute respiratory symptoms *[Likely, High Confidence]*."[42(p9)]

Increased Health Impacts from Wildfires

Key Finding: "Wildfires emit fine particles and ozone precursors that in turn increase the risk of premature death and adverse chronic and acute

---

[d] The report used the following scale for likelihood of occurrence: very likely, $\geq$ 9 in 10; likely, $\geq$ 2 in 3; as likely as not, $\approx$ 1 in 2; unlikely, $\leq$ 1 in 3; very unlikely, $\leq$ 1 in 10.[42(pXI)]

Figure 3 Framework Used by the Health Impacts of Climate Change Report

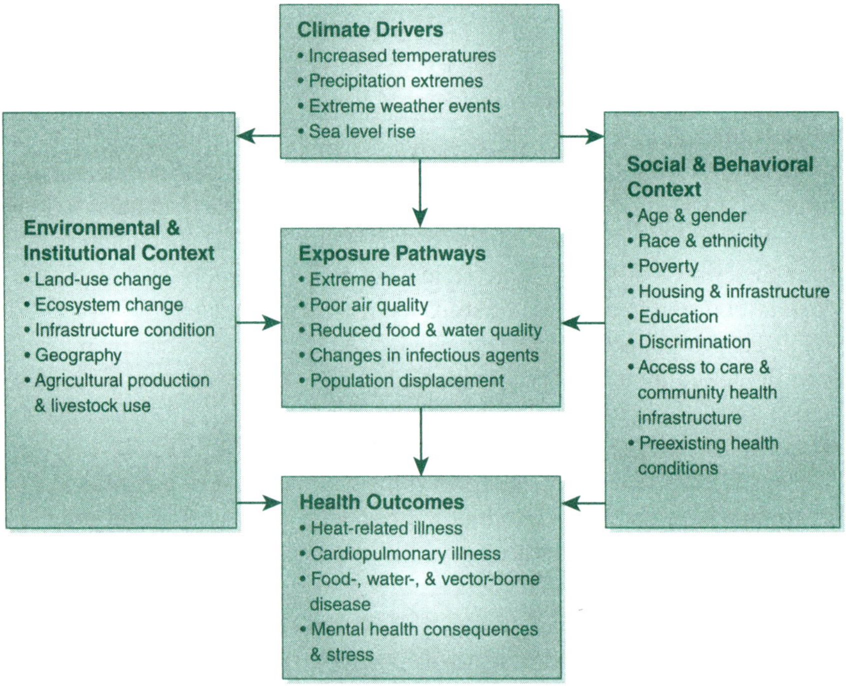

Conceptual diagram illustrating the exposure pathways by which climate change affects human health. Here, the center boxes list some selected examples of the kinds of changes in climate drivers, exposure, and health outcomes explored in the Health Impacts of Climate Change Report. Exposure pathways exist within the context of other factors that positively or negatively influence health outcomes (left-and right-side boxes). Some of the key factors that influence vulnerability for individuals are shown in the right box, and include social determinants of health and behavioral choices. Some key factors that influence vulnerability at larger scales, such as natural and built environments, governance and management, and institutions, are shown in the left box. All of these influencing factors can affect an individual's or a community's vulnerability through changes in exposure, sensitivity, and adaptive capacity and may also be affected by climate change.

Reproduced from Crimmins AJ, Balbus JL, Gamble CB, et al. Executive summary. In: *The Impacts of Climate Change on Human Health in the United States: A Scientific Assessment.* Washington, DC: U.S. Global Change Research Program; 2016:1–24. http://dx.doi.org/10.7930/J00P0WXS.

Table 1 Examples of Climate Impacts on Human Health

	Climate Driver	Exposure	Health Outcome	Impact
Extreme Heat	More frequent, severe, prolonged heat events	Elevated temperatures	Heat-related death and illness	Rising temperatures will lead to an increase in heat-related deaths and illnesses.
Outdoor Air Quality	Increasing temperatures and changing precipitation patterns	Worsened air quality (ozone, particulate matter, and higher pollen counts)	Premature death, acute and chronic cardiovascular and respiratory illnesses	Rising temperatures and wildfires and decreasing precipitation will lead to increases in ozone and particulate matter, elevating the risks of cardiovascular and respiratory illnesses and death.
Flooding	Rising sea level and more frequent or intense extreme precipitation, hurricanes, and storm surge events	Contaminated water, debris, and disruptions to essential infrastructure	Drowning, injuries, mental health consequences, gastrointestinal and other illness	Increased coastal and inland flooding exposes populations to a range of negative health impacts before, during, and after events.
Vector-Borne Infection (Lyme Disease)	Changes in temperature extremes and seasonal weather patterns	Earlier and geographically expanded tick activity	Lyme disease	Ticks will show earlier seasonal activity and a generally northward range expansion, increasing risk of human exposure to Lyme disease-causing bacteria.
Water-Related Infection (*Vibrio vulnificus*)	Rising sea surface temperature, changes in precipitation and runoff affecting coastal salinity	Recreational water or shellfish contaminated with *Vibrio vulnificus*	*Vibrio vulnificus*–induced diarrhea and intestinal illness,wound and blood-stream infections, death	Increases in water temperatures will alter timing and location of *Vibrio vulnificus* growth, increasing exposure and risk of waterborne illness.
Food-Related Infection (*Salmonella*)	Increases in temperature, humidity, and season length	Increased growth of pathogens, seasonal shifts in incidence of *Salmonella* exposure	*Salmonella* infection, gastrointestinal outbreaks	Rising temperatures increase *Salmonella* prevalence in food; longer seasons and warming winters increase risk of exposure and infection.
Mental Health and Well-Being	Climate change impacts, especially extreme weather	Level of exposure to traumatic events, like disasters	Distress, grief, behavioral health disorders, social impacts, resilience	Changes in exposure to climate- or weather-related disasters cause or exacerbate stress and mental health consequences, with greater risk for certain populations.

The table shows specific examples of how climate change can affect human health, now and in the future. These effects could occur at local, regional, or national scales. Moving from left to right along one health impact row, the three middle columns show how climate drivers affect an individual's or a community's exposure to a health threat and the resulting change in health outcome. The overall climate impact is summarized in the final column.

Reproduced from Crimmins AJ, Balbus JL, Gamble CB, et al. Executive summary. In: *The Impacts of Climate Change on Human Health in the United States: A Scientific Assessment.* Washington, DC: U.S. Global Change Research Program; 2016:1–24. http://dx.doi.org/10.7930/J00P0WXS.

cardiovascular and respiratory health outcomes *[Likely, High Confidence]*. Climate change is projected to increase the number and severity of naturally occurring wildfires in parts of the United States, increasing emissions of particulate matter and ozone precursors and resulting in additional adverse health outcomes *[Likely, High Confidence]*."[42(p9)]

Worsened Allergy and Asthma Conditions

Key Finding: "Changes in climate, specifically rising temperatures, altered precipitation patterns, and increasing concentrations of atmospheric carbon dioxide, are expected to contribute to increases in the levels of some airborne allergens and associated increases in asthma episodes and other allergic illnesses *[High Confidence]*."[42(p9)]

Changing Distributions of Vectors and Vector-Borne Diseases

Key Finding: "Climate change is expected to alter the geographic and seasonal distributions of existing vectors and vector-borne diseases *[Likely, High Confidence]*."[42(p13)]

Earlier Tick Activity and Northward Range Expansion

Key Finding: "Ticks capable of carrying the bacteria that cause Lyme disease and other pathogens will show earlier seasonal activity and a generally northward expansion in response to increasing temperatures associated with climate change *[Likely, High Confidence]*."[42(p13)]

Changing Mosquito-Borne Disease Dynamics

Key Finding: "Rising temperatures, changing precipitation patterns, and a higher frequency of some extreme weather events associated with climate change will influence the distribution, abundance, and prevalence of infection in the mosquitoes that transmit West Nile virus and other pathogens by altering habitat availability and mosquito and viral reproduction rates *[Very Likely, High Confidence]*."[42(p13)]

Emergence of New Vector-Borne Pathogens

Key Finding: "Vector-borne pathogens are expected to emerge or reemerge due to the interactions of climate factors with many other drivers, such as changing land-use patterns *[Likely, High Confidence]*. The impacts to human disease, however, will be limited by the adaptive capacity of human populations, such as vector control practices or personal protective measures *[Likely, High Confidence]*."[42(p13)]

These important and likely impacts of climate change illustrate the effects on humans. They also suggest One Health connections among human, animal, and ecosystem health.

We have now taken a look at the first two components of the One Health educational framework, which address the community and population impacts of microbiological influences as well as ecosystem changes. Now let us turn our attention to the final component, human–animal interactions, and examine both the positive and the negative impacts of these day-to-day interactions.

III. HUMAN–ANIMAL INTERACTIONS

Pet ownership is by far the most common way that most human beings come in contact with animals. There has been an estimated threefold increase in the number of dogs and cats owned as pets in the United States in the last half-century. Today nearly two-thirds of Americans own at least one pet. More than one-third of households have at least one dog and nearly one-third have at least one cat. In addition to the approximately 140 million pet dogs and cats in the United States, there are estimated to be approximately 5 million horses, 8 million birds, and more than 5 million small mammals plus a similar number of reptiles kept as pets.[43]

WHAT IS THE HUMAN–ANIMAL BOND AND WHAT ARE ITS HEALTH BENEFITS?

According to the American Veterinary Medical Association, the human–animal bond is "a mutually beneficial and dynamic relationship between people and animals that is influenced by behaviors that are essential to the health and well-being of both. This includes, but is not limited to, emotional, psychological, and physical interactions of people, animals, and the environment."[44]

The CDC recognizes the following benefits to human health from the interaction with pets:[45]

- Reduced blood pressure
- Reduced cholesterol and triglycerides
- Reduced feelings of loneliness
- Increased opportunities for exercise and outdoor activities
- Increased opportunities for socialization

The NIH News in Health provides some research evidence of the benefits of pet ownership. NIH indicates that:

> Some of the largest and most well-designed studies in this field suggest that four-legged friends can help to improve our cardiovascular health. One NIH-funded study looked at 421 adults who'd suffered heart attacks. A year later, the scientists found, dog owners were significantly more likely to still be alive than were those who did not own dogs, regardless of the severity of the heart attack.
>
> Another study looked at 240 married couples. Those who owned a pet were found to have lower heart rates and blood pressure, whether at rest or when undergoing stressful tests, than those without pets. Pet owners also seemed to have milder responses and quicker recovery from stress when they were with their pets than with a spouse or friend.
>
> The general belief is that there are health benefits to owning pets, both in terms of psychological growth and development, as well as physical health benefits.[46]

Evidence suggests additional benefits including reduced allergies and asthma among children exposed to pets during the first year of life and increased ability to communicate among children with autism.

Perhaps the best-studied and most well-publicized benefit of pet ownership has been the use of service animals, usually dogs. Service animals are now recognized as helpful not only to those with blindness and seizure disorders, but also to individuals with posttraumatic stress syndrome, as discussed in **Box 4**.

Although domesticated animals such as dogs and cats can provide considerable benefits to humans, they are not free of risk from zoonotic diseases.

WHAT ARE THE MAJOR RISKS FROM CATS AND DOGS AND HOW CAN THEY BE MINIMIZED?

Dogs and, to a lesser extent, cats are a potential source of rabies. Fortunately, proper vaccinations effectively protect dogs and cats as well as humans from this disease. The CDC recognizes a number of other preventable risks from cats and dogs including the following:

- Toxoplasmosis is an infection caused by a microscopic parasite called *Toxoplasma gondii*. Toxoplasmosis can cause severe illness in infants, including vision loss and seizures, when infected from their mothers before birth. The most common way for a pregnant woman to become infected is through contact with a cat's litter box. According to the

---

BOX 4 POSTTRAUMATIC STRESS DISORDER AND SERVICE ANIMALS

Posttraumatic stress disorder (PTSD) is an increasingly diagnosed condition, previously called shell shock and battle fatigue, which can develop in anyone after experiencing a severe traumatic event that threatens death or violence. Symptoms of PTSD continuing more than one month after the event often include the following manifestations:

- Flashbacks of the event
- Emotional isolation including avoidance of places that remind the individual of the traumatic event
- Hyperarousal including scanning for impending danger, sleep difficulties, and difficulties with concentration and outbursts of anger
- Negativity and guilt, often accompanied by headaches, heart palpitations, and feelings of dizziness, as well as a lack of interest in other people, even close family members

A range of studies suggest that companion animals, usually trained service dogs, can improve many of these symptoms. For instance, the presence of an animal may act as a comforting reminder that danger is no longer present. The presence of an animal has been reported to elicit positive emotions and warmth. Animals can also serve as social facilitators that can help connect with people and reduce loneliness. Pets, unlike humans, are nonjudgmental and offer outward signs of unconditional love and affection on an ongoing basis. Consequently, sufferers of PTSD may find it easier to be around animals than to be in the company of people.[47,48]

PTSD research continues but service dogs are already being widely used and accepted as part of PSTD treatment.

CDC, pregnant women ideally should avoid changing a cat's litter box and avoid adopting stray cats. Everyone should cover outdoor sandboxes to keep animals away.[49]

- Cat-scratch disease (CSD) is a bacterial infection spread by cats. The disease spreads when an infected cat licks a person's open wound or bites or scratches a person hard enough to break the surface of the skin, often leading to spread of the infection to the lymph nodes. Washing cat bites and scratches well with soap and running water helps prevent human disease. People should not allow cats to lick human wounds. Approximately 40% of cats carry the disease-producing bacteria *Bartonella henselae* at some time in their lives, although most cats with this infection show no signs of illness.[50]

A wide range of bacterial diseases can be transmitted by cats and dogs and require caution, especially when disposing of feces. Perhaps the most serious disease transmitted to humans by dogs (and far less frequently by cats) is toxocariasis, which the CDC has identified as a "neglected parasitic infection in the United States," one of a group of diseases that results in significant illness among those who are infected and is often poorly understood by healthcare providers.

Toxocariasis is a preventable parasitic infection caused by the larval form of the dog or cat roundworms *Toxocara canis* and *Toxocara cati*. *Toxocara* eggs are often found in dog feces and occasionally cat feces. People can acquire toxocariasis if they accidentally come in skin contact with or ingest dirt containing *Toxocara* eggs after gardening or playing in dirt or sand contaminated with infected feces. After skin contact with the *Toxocara* eggs, the larvae hatch and may travel under the skin (cutaneous larva migrans or creeping eruption). Rarely, toxocariasis can invade the eyes and other organs including the brain, where it can cause severe damage. Preventive measures greatly reduce the risk of developing toxocariasis. These measures commonly include controlling *Toxocara* infection in dogs through deworming by a veterinarian and reducing contact with the larvae by promptly disposing of dog and cat feces to a place away from people.[51]

The preventable diseases caused by cats and dogs are viewed by most Americans as far less of a threat than the many benefits of the human–animal bond. The same cannot be said of other types of pets that the CDC has called "exotic pets."

WHAT IS MEANT BY EXOTIC PETS AND WHAT RISKS DO THEY POSE FOR INFECTIOUS DISEASE?

There are approximately 10 million animals imported into the United States each year, including amphibians, birds, mammals, and reptiles. Check out the Internet and you will see that included in these numbers is a thriving trade in what has been called exotic species. Exotic species are non-native species including many large and small animals not found in the United States. For most of these animals, except for nonhuman primates, there are no federal requirements for disease screening. Exotic pets also include native species of reptiles and amphibians. Debate has arisen over whether domestic small mammals, many of which can carry diseases transmittable to humans, should be considered as exotic species.[52]

According to *National Geographic*, "in Americans' backyards and garages and living rooms, in their beds and basements and bathrooms, wild animals kept as pets live side by side with their human owners. It's believed that more exotic animals live in American homes than are cared for in American zoos…. Privately owning exotic animals is currently permitted in a handful of states with essentially no restrictions: You must have a license to own a dog, but you are free to purchase a lion or baboon and keep it as a pet."[53]

Animals imported for commercial trade represent a substantial risk to human health. For instance, monkeypox, a less severe disease related to smallpox, was introduced into the United States when a shipment of African Gambian giant rats was sold to dealers, one of whom housed the rats with prairie dogs intended for sale as pets. The prairie dogs subsequently became ill and transmitted the infection to 71 people, including prairie dog owners and veterinary staff caring for the ill animals. Less headline grabbing but no less important is the common occurrence of *Salmonella* outbreaks posed by domestic reptiles such as small turtles.[53,54]

The risks posed by exotic pet ownership illustrate the components of One Health. That is, exotic pet ownership illustrates the risk that these animals pose to the ecosystem as well as to human health. For example, pet pythons that have been released into wetlands have become unchecked predators. Lionfish, an invasive marine species common in the aquarium trade, are now threatening reefs throughout the Caribbean and Gulf of Mexico due to their release into the ocean by pet owners in Florida.[55]

We have now completed our look at the microbiological threats, the impact of ecosystem change, and the impacts of close human–animal interactions on health. Throughout this discussion we have suggested ways to encourage healthier and more sustainable interactions among humans, animals, and the environment. However, it is also important to take a big-picture look at what can be done to address the major risks to human populations, especially from emerging and reemerging infectious diseases with potential for epidemic and pandemic spread.

ONE HEALTH: PUTTING IT INTO PRACTICE

One Health addresses a wide spectrum of health consequences ranging from infectious diseases to allergies, cancer, and mental health. Our discussion of the components of One Health suggests a number of general approaches to reduce the risks associated with the interactions among humans, animals, and the ecosystem:

- Efforts to minimize the extent of climate change
- Attention to the impacts of "industrial" production of animal products
- Control of human exposure to exotic pets
- Judicious use of antibiotics in humans and animals
- Better communication and collaboration among human, animal, and environmental health professionals

Perhaps the most feared human health impacts relate to epidemic and potentially pandemic diseases. Therefore we focus our attention on epidemic and pandemic infectious disease as we examine what can be done to put One Health into practice.

WHAT CAN BE DONE TO PREVENT AND CONTROL THE EPIDEMIC AND PANDEMIC SPREAD OF HUMAN COMMUNICABLE DISEASES?

A number of interventions can be undertaken to prevent, detect, and control the epidemic and pandemic spread of communicable diseases. These might be thought of as the five Ss of control of communicable diseases.

1. Surveillance—active human monitoring of emerging and reemerging diseases, especially RNA viral diseases, is needed in areas with high biodiversity and/or where large numbers of people interact with a diversity of both wild and domestic animal species.[e] Active surveillance may be key to successful efforts to institute early response and control measures.
2. Spillover investigations—when new diseases emerging from animals are first detected in humans, these spillover diseases warrant especially close monitoring and investigations of additional populations to ensure that the disease does not acquire the ability to be transmitted from person to person.
3. Sentinel investigation—monitoring of specific animal species for increases in disease frequency may serve as an early warning sign of

---

[e] Areas with high biodiversity include sub-Saharan Africa, Southeast Asia, and the Amazon basin. The markets of southeastern China are an example of a location where humans interact frequently with both wild and domestic animal species.

increased human transmission as has been done for West Nile virus for selected species of birds.

4. Statistics—Once an emerging virus is detected in human populations, high-quality and "real-time" statistics are needed to monitor and guide attempts to limit its spread to new populations.
5. Studies—research into new vaccines, drugs, and other technological approaches needs to be an ongoing effort, not merely a response to an emergency.

Even with these types of actions, human beings will remain threatened by public health emergencies caused by pandemic disease.

WHAT CAN BE DONE TO RESPOND TO THE THREAT OF PANDEMIC DISEASES?

Pandemic disease, by definition, requires more than a national response; it requires a global response. Epidemic and widespread pandemics have occurred since ancient times, yet until the late 19th century there was little or no coordinated international response to such events. The International Sanitary Convention of 1892, the first such international effort, focused attention on a subset of diseases, primarily cholera, plague, and yellow fever, and the quarantine regulations necessary to prevent the shipping trade from transporting these diseases across international borders.

The WHO was established as a United Nations organization in 1948. In 1951, WHO adopted the existing agreements as the International Health Regulations (IHR), which became binding on all WHO members. These regulations were limited to cholera, plague, yellow fever, and smallpox, with smallpox being removed from the IHR after its eradication in the late 1970s.

Public health emergencies of the 21st century were required before the international community succeeded in modernizing the IHR. In 2005, after the SARS epidemic, the IHR was modified in a number of important ways.[56–58]

- The scope of the IHR (2005) was expanded with the intent to protect against, control, and provide a public health response to the international spread of disease.
- The IHR (2005) embraced an all-hazards strategy, covering health threats irrespective of their origin or source, as opposed to the previous disease-specific coverage. The intention was to include biological, chemical, and nuclear events.

- The IHR (2005) requires nations to develop core capacities for rapid detection, assessment, reporting, and response to potential "public health emergencies of international concern," including surveillance, laboratories, and risk communication. Core capacities are central to a public health strategy of strengthening local infrastructure and systems to detect and contain outbreaks at their source before they spread internationally.

- To be in compliance with the IHR, member countries were required to promptly notify WHO of events that might constitute a public health emergency of international concern, with a continuing obligation to inform WHO of any updates.

- On the basis of information from nations (official sources) or from unofficial sources, WHO's director general was authorized to declare a "public health emergency of international concern" (PHEIC). Declaration of a PHEIC allows WHO to make unbinding disease control recommendations, provide assistance, and communicate with other nations regarding the health threat.

Public health emergencies of international concern were declared by the WHO director for the influenza pandemic of 2009–2010 as well as for the Ebola epidemic of 2014–2015, and most recently for the Zika epidemic in February 2016.

The Ebola epidemic, like the SARS epidemic, created enormous worldwide fear and eventually major international responses. One impact of the Ebola epidemic was the creation of the Commission on a Global Health Risk Framework for the Future,[f] which was developed to provide advice on how the international community should react to future public health emergencies.[59]

The commission described the Ebola epidemic as follows:

> With failures occurring at all levels, the recent Ebola outbreak in West Africa exposed significant weaknesses in the global health system and culminated in a tragic humanitarian disaster. At the national level in affected countries, there was significant delay in acknowledging the magnitude of the outbreak. And after the outbreak was recognized,

---

[f] The commission was an independent group of 17 international experts from 12 countries overseen by "eminent and diverse leaders" from Africa, Asia, Europe, and the Americas and supported by many of the world's largest private foundations, including the Gates Foundation and the Wellcome Trust, as well as by the U.S. Agency for International Development.

the international response was slow and uncoordinated. Mechanisms for the establishment of public–private partnerships were lacking. For example, the development of lifesaving medical products was reactive, rather than proactive. An easily mobilized reserve of funds to support the response was not available. Critical financial and human resources were slow to arrive or never arrived at all. Countries were reluctant to acknowledge the severity of the outbreak and obstructed early notification. Surveillance and information systems were not in place or failed to provide early warning.[59(p9)]

The commission argued that public health emergencies should be viewed in light of their potential economic costs and their impact on global security, not solely as health issues. It made specific recommendations with a short timeline for action in three areas. First, the commission recommended reinforcing national public health capabilities and infrastructure as the first line of defense against potential pandemics. Second, the commission recommended more effective global and regional capabilities led by a reenergized WHO, through a dedicated Center for Health Emergency Preparedness and Response (CHEPR) designed to coordinate effectively with the rest of the UN system, as well as the World Bank and International Monetary Fund (IMF). Finally, the commission recommended an accelerated WHO-led research and development effort coordinated by an independent Pandemic Product Development Committee (PPDC) to mobilize, prioritize, allocate, and oversee research and development resources relating to infectious diseases with pandemic potential.

The commission did not recommend changing the basic legal framework of the 2005 International Health Regulations. Rather, it recommended a series of changes in IHR procedures plus new funding and authority to better position the international and national communities to respond to future public health emergencies of international concern.

Table 2 summarizes and compares the International Health Regulations as they existed from 1951 until 2007, when the IHR (2005) was implemented, as well as the additional changes recommended by the commission.

In the 21st century, the international community has begun to respond to the threat of pandemic disease by strengthening the role of the WHO and other international organizations as well as by attempting to ensure sufficient local capacities. This process will require continuing modifications and enhancements if the world expects to effectively control emerging infections and prevent pandemic diseases.

Table 2 International Health Regulations Changes

	1951–2007	2007–Present	Proposed by Commission
Scope	Cholera, plague, yellow fever, smallpox (removed after eradication) Control at borders/ports	Required reporting of public health emergency of international concern—not limited to infectious disease Detection and containment at source	Additional reporting of watch list of outbreaks with potential to become a public health emergency of international concern
WHO Authority	WHO could not initiate an inquiry	WHO can initiate an inquiry based on "unofficial sources" and can ask for additional information from "official sources." WHO director can declare a public health emergency of international concern	WHO would also have authority over a watch list of outbreaks
Expectations of Member States/Nations	Defined capacities at ports	Set of minimum core capacities for detection, reporting, and assessment with self-reporting of capacities	Require external assessment of core capacities with use of "name and share" to encourage compliance
Consequence of Noncompliance with Reporting Requirements and Implementation of Core Capacities	No formal consequences or required external assessment of core capacities	No formal consequences or required external assessment of core capacities	International Monetary Fund and World Bank take noncompliance and pandemic preparedness into account in their economic and policy assessment of nations

(continues)

	1951–2007	2007–Present	Proposed by Commission
Coordination of Response	No mechanism for coordination of response	WHO expected to provide assistance in response, communicate with other nations, and recommend control measures	Release of financial resources from WHO emergency funds and World Bank resources
International Response Capabilities	Set of predetermined controls limited to borders and ports	Flexible evidence-based responses adapted to nature of the threat	Greater technical assistance and scientific advice including funds for research and development (PPDC)

SUMMARY

We have now taken a look at the origins and goals of the One Health movement, which focuses on the connections among human health, animal health, and health of the ecosystem. We began by acknowledging the wide range of microbiological entities that can produce human disease. RNA viruses represent a large percentage of the emerging diseases, especially those capable of producing pandemic disease. We also discussed a set of top 10 RNA viruses chosen to reflect the scope of the threats that humans face from RNA viruses.

Ecosystem change underlies many of the threats we face, but also illustrates the opportunities to improve health of all humans—not just those with the resources to respond effectively to ecosystem change. We can organize an approach to ecosystem change using a framework addressing global movements of populations, agriculture and changes in food distribution, ecological changes in land and resource use, technological changes that affect the ecosystem, and climate change.

Another component of our examination of One Health focused on the interactions between humans and animals. Pets, especially dogs and cats, often provide benefits through the human–animal bond, and dogs can often be specially trained to function as service animals. The most important human diseases caused by dogs and cats are preventable or controllable.

Exotic pets, including domestic as well as imported animals, pose much greater risks to humans.

The One Health framework suggests a range of options to prevent and control infectious disease, including what we have called the five Ss of control of communicable disease. Global cooperation, however, is needed to detect and control potential pandemic disease. The International Health Regulations represent a framework for global cooperation but require ongoing enhancement and modification to address the continuing and emerging threats of pandemic disease.

ACKNOWLEDGMENTS

The authors would like to acknowledge the invaluable assistance provided by the following two reviewers:

Bernadette Dunham, DVM, PhD, former Director, Center for Veterinary Medicine, U.S. Food and Drug Administration

Claire Standley, PhD, MSc, Assistant Professor, Department of International Health, Georgetown University

Their careful review of a draft of this text was of great assistance in ensuring the accuracy and clarity of the material. However, any errors or lack of clarity are the sole responsibility of the authors.

REFERENCES

1. American Association of Veterinary Medical Colleges. One Health Educational Framework for health professional students. http://www.aavmc.org/One-Health/Case-Studies.aspx. Accessed June 27, 2016.
2. Centers for Disease Control and Prevention. A history of anthrax. http://www.cdc.gov/anthrax/resources/history. Accessed June 27, 2016.
3. Centers for Disease Control and Prevention. Rabies. http://www.cdc.gov/rabies/index.html. Accessed June 27, 2016.
4. Centers for Disease Control and Prevention. *Mycobacterium bovis* (bovine tuberculosis) in humans. http://www.cdc.gov/tb/publications/factsheets/general/mbovis.htm. Accessed June 27, 2016.
5. Trichinella.org. *Trichinella* history: part 2: discovery of the life cycle. http://www.trichinella.org/history_2.htm. Accessed June 27, 2016.
6. Schultz M. Photo quiz: Rudolph Virchow. *Emerg Infect Dis* [serial online]. 2008. 14(9):1480–1481. doi: 10.3201/eid1409.086672.

7. Reed LD. A message from the editor. *Public Health Rep.* 2008;123(3):257.
8. Lederberg J. Infectious history. *Science.* 2000;288(5464):287–293. doi: 10.1126/science.288.5464.287.
9. Kahn RE, Clouser DF, Richt JA. Emerging infections: a tribute to the one medicine, one health concept. *Zoonoses Public Health.* 2009;56:407–428. doi: 10.1111/j.1863-2378.2009.01255.x.
10. Cardiff RD, Ward JM, Barthold SW. "One medicine—one pathology": are veterinary and human pathology prepared? *Lab Investig.* 2008;88:18–26.
11. One Health Initiative. One Health Initiative will unite human and veterinary medicine. http://www.onehealthinitiative.com. Accessed June 27, 2016.
12. Woolhouse MEJ, Adair K, Brierley L. RNA viruses: a case study of the biology of emerging infectious diseases. *Microbiol Spectr.* 2013;1(1):OH-0001-2012. doi: 10.1128/microbiolspec.OH-0001-2012.
13. Wolfe ND, Dunavan CP, Diamond J. Origins of major human infectious diseases. *Nature.* 2007;447:279–283. doi: 10.1038/nature05775.
14. De Cock KM, Jaffe HW, Curran JW. Reflections on 30 years of AIDS. *Emerg Infect Dis* [serial online]. 2011;17(6):1044–1048. doi: 10.3201/eid/1706.100184.
15. Centers for Disease Control and Prevention. Chikungunya virus. http://www.cdc.gov/chikungunya. Accessed June 27, 2016.
16. Centers for Disease Control and Prevention. Dengue. Frequently asked questions. http://www.cdc.gov/dengue/faqfacts/index.html. Accessed July 19, 2016.
17. Centers for Disease Control and Prevention. Dengue. http://www.cdc.gov/dengue/index.html. Accessed June 27, 2016.
18. World Health Organization. Dengue and severe dengue. http://www.who.int/mediacentre/factsheets/fs117/en. Accessed June 27, 2016.
19. Centers for Disease Control and Prevention. Ebola (Ebola virus disease). http://www.cdc.gov/vhf/ebola/index.html. Accessed June 27, 2016.
20. Centers for Disease Control and Prevention. Hantavirus. http://www.cdc.gov/hantavirus. Accessed June 27, 2016.
21. Barcott B. Death at Yosemite: the story behind last summer's hantavirus outbreak. *Outside.* December 18, 2012. http://www.outsideonline.com/1930876/death-yosemite-story-behind-last-summers-hantavirus-outbreak. Accessed June 27, 2016.
22. Centers for Disease Control and Prevention. Influenza (flu). http://www.cdc.gov/flu. Accessed June 27, 2016.
23. Centers for Disease Control and Prevention. Middle East respiratory syndrome (MERS). http://www.cdc.gov/coronavirus/mers/about/index.html. Accessed June 27, 2016.
24. Boyer L. Stop drinking camel urine, World Health Organization says. *U.S. News & World Report.* June 10, 2015. http://www.usnews.com/news/articles/2015/06/10/stop-drinking-camel-urine-world-health-organization-says. Accessed June 27, 2016.
25. Bradsher K, Altman LK. China to kill 10,000 civet cats in effort to eradicate SARS. *New York Times.* January 5, 2004. http://www.nytimes.com/2004/01/05/world/china-to-kill-10000-civet-cats-in-effort-to-eradicate-sars.html?_r=0. Accessed June 27, 2016.

26. Koplan JP, Butler-Jones D, Tsang T, Yu W. Public health lessons from severe acute respiratory syndrome a decade later. *Emerg Infect Dis* [serial online]. 2013;19(6): 861–863. doi: 10.3201/eid1906.121426.

27. Centers for Disease Control and Prevention. West Nile virus. http://www.cdc.gov /westnile. Accessed June 27, 2016.

28. World Health Organization. The history of Zika virus. http://www.who.int/emergencies /zika-virus/history/en. Accessed June 27, 2016.

29. Centers for Disease Control and Prevention. Zika virus. http://www.cdc.gov/zika /symptoms. Accessed June 27, 2016.

30. Morse SS. Factors in the emergence of infectious diseases. *Emerg Infect Dis* [serial online]. 1995;1(1):7–15. doi: 10.3201/eid0101.950102.

31. Morens DM, Folkers GK, Fauci AS. Emerging infections: a perpetual challenge. *Lancet Infect Dis.* 2008;8:710–719. doi: 10.1016/S1473-3099(08)70256-1.

32. Coker R, Rushton J, Mounier-Jack S, et al. Towards a conceptual framework to support one-health research for policy on emerging zoonoses. *Lancet Infect Dis.* 2011;11(4):326–331. doi: 10.1016/S1473-3099(10)70312-1.

33. Entis L.Will the worst bird flu outbreak in US history finally make us reconsider factory farming chicken? *The Guardian.* July 14, 2015. http://www.theguardian.com /vital-signs/2015/jul/14/bird-flu-devastation-highlights-unsustainability-of-commercial -chicken-farming. Accessed June 27, 2016.

34. Goldsmith E, Hildyard N. Dams and disease. January 1, 1984. http://www.edwardgoldsmith .org/1018/dams-and-disease. Accessed June 27, 2016.

35. Centers for Disease Control and Prevention. Lyme disease. http://www.cdc.gov/lyme. Accessed June 27, 2016.

36. Centers for Disease Control and Prevention. Haiti cholera outbreak. http://www.cdc .gov/haiticholera/haiti_cholera.htm. Accessed June 27, 2016.

37. Centers for Disease Control and Prevention. Parasites—American trypanosomiasis (also known as Chagas disease). http://www.cdc.gov/parasites/chagas/gen_info/detailed .html. Accessed June 27, 2016.

38. U.S. Environmental Protection Agency. International actions: The Montreal Proto-col on Substances That Deplete the Ozone Layer. https://www.epa.gov/ozone-layer -protection/international-actions-montreal-protocol-substances-deplete-ozone-layer. Accessed June 27, 2016.

39. Centers for Disease Control and Prevention. About antimicrobial resistance. http:// www.cdc.gov/drugresistance/about.html. Accessed June 27, 2016.

40. U.S. Food and Drug Administration. FDA reminds retail establishments of upcoming changes to the use of antibiotics in food animals. June 20, 2016. http://www.fda.gov /AnimalVeterinary/NewsEvents/CVMUpdates/ucm507355.htm. Accessed June 27, 2016.

41. Centers for Disease Control and Prevention. National strategy to combat antibiotic-resistant bacteria. http://www.cdc.gov/drugresistance/federal-engagement-in-ar/national-strategy/index.html. Accessed June 27, 2016.

42. Crimmins AJ, Balbus JL, Gamble CB, et al. *The Impacts of Climate Change on Human Health in the United States: A Scientific Assessment.* Washington, DC: U.S. Global Change Research Program; 2016. http://dx.doi.org/10.7930/J00P0WXS.

43. American Veterinary Medical Association. U.S. pet ownership statistics. https://www.avma.org/KB/Resources/Statistics/Pages/Market-research-statistics-US-pet-ownership.aspx. Accessed June 27, 2016.

44. American Veterinary Medical Association. Human–animal bond. https://www.avma.org/kb/resources/reference/human-animal-bond/pages/human-animal-bond-avma.aspx. Accessed June 27, 2016.

45. Centers for Disease Control and Prevention. Healthy pets healthy people. http://www.cdc.gov/healthypets. Accessed June 27, 2016.

46. National Institutes of Health. Can pets help keep you healthy? Exploring the human-animal bond. *NIH News in Health.* February 2009:1–2. https://newsinhealth.nih.gov/2009/February/feature1.htm. Accessed June 27, 2016.

47. O'Haire ME, Guérin NA, Kirkham AC. Animal-Assisted Intervention for trauma: a systematic literature review. *Front Psychol* [serial online]. 2015;6:1121. doi: 10.3389/fpsyg.2015.01121.

48. WebMD. Posttraumatic stress disorder. http://www.webmd.com/mental-health/post-traumatic-stress-disorder. Accessed June 27, 2016.

49. Centers for Disease Control and Prevention. Parasites: toxoplasmosis (*Taxoplasma* infection). http://www.cdc.gov/parasites/toxoplasmosis. Accessed June 1, 2016.

50. Centers for Disease Control and Prevention. Cat-scratch disease. http://www.cdc.gov/healthypets/diseases/cat-scratch.html. Accessed June 27, 2016.

51. Centers for Disease Control and Prevention. Parasites: toxocariasis (also known as roundworm infection). http://www.cdc.gov/parasites/toxocariasis. Accessed June 27, 2016.

52. Marano N, Arguin PM, Pappaioanou M. Impact of globalization and animal trade on infectious disease ecology. *Emerg Infect Dis* [serial online]. 2007;13(12):1807–1809. doi: 10.3201/eid1312.071276.

53. Slater L. Exotic pets. *National Geographic.* April 2014. http://ngm.nationalgeographic.com/2014/04/exotic-pets/slater-text. Accessed June 27, 2016.

54. U.S. Food and Drug Administration. *Pet Turtles: Cute But Commonly Contaminated with Salmonella.* Silver Spring, MD: U.S. Food and Drug Administration; 2016. http://www.fda.gov/downloads/ForConsumers/ConsumerUpdates/UCM203088.pdf. Accessed June 27, 2016.

55. World Resource Institute. Atlantic and Caribbean: lionfish invasion threatens reefs. http://www.wri.org/atlantic-and-caribbean-lionfish-invasion-threatens-reefs. Accessed June 27, 2016.

56. Gostin LO, DeBartolo MC, Friedman EA. The International Health Regulations 10 years on: the governing framework for global health security. *Lancet.* 2015;386(10009): 2222–2226.

57. Katz R, Fischer J. The revised International Health Regulations: a framework for global pandemic response. *Global Health Governance.* 2010;3(2). https://www.researchgate .net/publication/264868835_The_Revised_International_Health_Regulations_A _Framework_for_Global_Pandemic_Response. Accessed June 27, 2016.

58. World Health Organization. Alert, response, and capacity building under the International Health Regulations (IHR). http://www.who.int/ihr/about/10things/en. Accessed June 27, 2016.

59. GHRF Commission (Commission on a Global Health Risk Framework for the Future). *The Neglected Dimension of Global Security: A Framework to Counter Infectious Disease Crises.* Washington, DC: Commission on a Global Health Risk Framework for the Future; 2016. http://www.nap.edu/catalog/21891/the-neglected-dimension-of -global-security-a-framework-to-counter. Accessed June 27, 2016.